MHAMEAMA

50 Healthy Tips for Women with PCOS

A Guide to a well-Balanced Healthy Habit for women living with Polycystic Ovarian Syndrome

Copyright © 2024 by MhameAma

All rights reserved. No part of this publication may be reproduced, stored or transmitted in any form or by any means, electronic, mechanical, photocopying, recording, scanning, or otherwise without written permission from the publisher. It is illegal to copy this book, post it to a website, or distribute it by any other means without permission.

MhameAma asserts the moral right to be identified as the author of this work.

MhameAma has no responsibility for the persistence or accuracy of URLs for external or third-party Internet Websites referred to in this publication and does not guarantee that any content on such Websites is, or will remain, accurate or appropriate.

Designations used by companies to distinguish their products are often claimed as trademarks. All brand names and product names used in this book and on its cover are trade names, service marks, trademarks and registered trademarks of their respective owners. The publishers and the book are not associated with any product or vendor mentioned in this book. None of the companies referenced within the book have endorsed the book.

First edition

This book was professionally typeset on Reedsy.
Find out more at reedsy.com

I am dedicating this book to all of the women out there who, in some way, lean into their body insecurities and tell themselves, "I am not good enough." I want you to know that you are MORE THAN ENOUGH, SUPER WOMAN!

When dreams come true, desires fade away.

-A MUSICIAN QUOTE

Contents

1

Introduction

Step right into the world of "50 Healthy Tips for PCOS Women." This book is more than just a list of rules; it serves as a guiding light, a path to strength, and a tribute to the perseverance of women facing Polycystic Ovarian Syndrome (PCOS).

I am one of those brave and resilient women who refuse to let PCOS define us. My arduous journey with Polycystic Ovary Syndrome has been filled with countless inescapable challenges, overwhelming frustrations, and heart-wrenching moments of despair. However, amidst the darkness, a flickering flame of hope has persisted.

Throughout this arduous battle, I have understood that knowledge is truly empowering. Armed with information and awareness, we can reshape our destinies. Taking proactive steps towards managing PCOS can create a seismic shift in our lives, etching a profound and lasting impact.

Although the road ahead may appear daunting, I am determined to conquer this condition. I refuse to surrender to its debilitating grip. Instead, I rally the courage to uplift others grappling with the same trials. Together, we can amass a formidable force of resilience and determination.

Thus, let us embark on an expedition towards triumph. Let us become warriors armed with wisdom and equipped with invaluable tools to combat PCOS. As we navigate this uncharted terrain, we will unearth hidden strengths and cultivate a tenacious spirit to guide us through even the darkest times.

Remember, my fellow PCOS warriors, we are not defined by our diagnoses. We are defined by our unwavering strength, refusal to be defeated, and relentless pursuit of a brighter future. Together, we can break the chains that bind us and emerge victorious champions in adversity.

Within the pages of this publication, I not only present scientifically backed methodologies but also offer intimate perspectives and individual encounters. Working in tandem, we will delve into the intricate components of managing PCOS, from dietary intake and physical activity to stress mitigation and reproductive well-being.

I invite you to accompany me on this expedition of enlightenment, empowerment, and personal well-being. Together, we shall equip ourselves with wisdom, assist one another, and adopt a harmonious, healthy routine to nurture our physical, mental, and spiritual well-being.

General Overview

Polycystic ovary syndrome (PCOS) was first described in 1935 by Stein, Levental, and Barg, who found that the signs are associated with the presence of polycystic ovaries. The cause of PCOS has not been identified due to the inability to perform a severe test of chemo-endocrine function in sequential samples of everyday women and women with these syndromes. An abnormal cycle of pituitary and ovarian hormone secretion is thought to be the cause of the disease. Specifically, PCOS is a syndrome of androgen excess.

Due to insulin resistance and increasing obesity, PCOS is associated with other pathologies such as hyperandrogenism, chronic anovulation and infertility, hyperlipidemia, hypertension, and type 2 diabetes mellitus. This syndrome affects 5–10% of women of reproductive age. Since its first identification, PCOS has been diagnosed frequently, and many of its mysterious signs slowly finally receive an explanation. In general, whatever the views on PCOS, these patients need reliable health tips.

Attention to the health and wellness of polycystic ovary syndrome (PCOS) primarily focuses on weight loss and insulin resistance monitoring. Dietary advice is prescribed to control and reduce weight. The recommendation of anti-diabetic drugs and in vitro fertilization (IVF) also needs weight reduction. The unique characteristic of PCOS is menstrual irregularity or anovulatory cycles. Underweight or overweight conditions could disrupt this, and energy requirements are at the bottom. As complicated as it is, dietary advice sporadically depends on energy needs alone. 'Healthy' nutritional patterns are similarly popular among PCOS; thus, the different contradictions and uniqueness of PCOS require constant attention and individualization for improvement of the syndrome. As an endocrine syndrome, the treatment is more than dietary advice. Therefore, this review was done to summarize recent health tips specifically for women with PCOS. 2

1.1. Definition and Symptoms of PCOS

What is polycystic ovary syndrome (PCOS)?

Polycystic ovary syndrome (PCOS) is a hormonal disorder common among women of reproductive age. Women with PCOS may have infrequent or prolonged menstrual periods or excess male hormone (androgen) levels. The ovaries may develop numerous small collections of fluid (follicles) and fail to release eggs regularly.

What are the symptoms of PCOS?

Symptoms tend to be mild at first. You may have only a few symptoms or a lot of them. The most common symptoms are: Acne is a common skin condition that can cause pimples and blemishes on the face, chest, back, or buttocks. Another symptom associated with excessive hair growth, known as hirsutism, is unwanted hair in these areas. In addition to these physical changes, individuals may also experience thinning hair on the scalp, which can be distressing for many. Irregular periods are yet another common symptom that can disrupt a woman's reproductive health, making it more challenging to conceive. Lastly, obesity and infertility can also be linked to these hormonal imbalances, highlighting the multifactorial nature of this condition. It is essential to seek medical advice and explore treatment options if you are experiencing any of these symptoms, as early intervention can help manage the effects of this complex disorder.

1.2. Prevalence and Impact on Women's Health

PCOS is the most common endocrine disorder in premenopausal women and affects approximately 7–20% of reproductive-aged women. The existence of its features in women with numerous different racial and ethnic backgrounds suggests that its etiology may be both complex and diverse within the individual patient. The health implications of PCOS are all-encompassing and could result in quite burdensome medical and diagnostic expenses for the same. It may also cause significant premature death and a total loss of productivity across the lifespan. Women with PCOS face a life course spent worrying about fertility loss, future diabetes, sexual problems, obesity, eating disorders, cancer, and other significant chronic diseases. Yet the harsh fact is that many physicians, the funders involved, and far too many women with the syndrome have limited or no direct knowledge of its effects on female reproductive health, especially during their childbearing period.

1.3. Importance of Lifestyle Management for PCOS

We aren't managing the problem (PCOS), and we aren't helping women develop healthier relationships with food and natural ways to combat insulin. It is important to remember that the cornerstone of PCOS management is lifestyle management. Not just with foods but with sleep, stress, environmental endocrine disruptors, exercise, and realizing that our day-to-day food intake doesn't just affect our blood glucose levels and the body's fat tissue, which is an endocrine organ in and of itself. By consuming only a tiny bit too much glucose, or any food for that matter, women with PCOS may be negatively affecting their hormonal milieu by disrupting hormone receptors and by blocking the normal reproductive and endocrine function of ovarian tissue, which can lead to very high insulin levels and inflammation both in the ovary and systemically. Women with PCOS must also factor in how any small dietary indiscretion can rapidly translate into a significant increase in their insulin levels. This altered hormone environment then sets women with PCOS up for an increased risk for health problems such as infertility, cardiovascular disease, abnormal lipid profiles, and type 2 diabetes.

The cornerstone of polycystic ovary syndrome (PCOS) management is lifestyle management. For instance, in the United States, asking your average registered dietitian for advice on PCOS all too often results in being told to eat a diet high in whole grains. Why? A diet high in whole grains has decreased the risk of type 2 diabetes. And women with PCOS have an increased risk of type 2 diabetes, as do men with PCOS. That's all well and good, but focusing on whole grains in a diet is not treating the underlying disease of PCOS or its significant symptoms of irregular menstrual cycles and infertility.

2

Nutrition and Diet Tips

Consume healthy fats in sesame, seeds, walnuts, and walnut oil. Fats are also crucial for the proper functioning of the body. They are an energy source, help absorb certain vitamins and minerals, make our cells healthy and produce certain vital hormones. But do not consume excessive quantities. Choose feta cheese, ricotta cheese, paneer, and low-fat cheese. The amount of fat intake, especially saturated fats, is crucial for the diet of PCOS patients. It has been proven that high levels of long-chain saturated fats are associated with insulin resistance in women with PCOS.

Choose fat-free proteins such as lentils, chickpeas, black beans, fava beans, kidney beans, black-eyed peas, mung beans, lima beans, perdu beans, fava beans, white beans, and broad beans. Proteins are the building blocks of all cells, tissues, and organs. So, they are essential in the development of a fetus. Our hair and nails are made of protein. Our body also uses proteins to make hemoglobin, which enables the transport of nutrients, hormones, and oxygen to all our cells. Proteins are found in dairy, soy, eggs, meat, and fish products, and fish and meat are richer in protein. Choose those with a high percentage of fat-free protein and do not consume excessive quantities.

2.1. Balanced Diet Recommendations

1. Fill half your plate with vegetables. Limiting high-carb foods like bread, rice, pasta, and sugary foods, bulk up on non-starchy vegetables such as broccoli, leafy greens, mushrooms, onions, cauliflower, and bell peppers. Make sure to switch up these veggies and aim to eat a variety to amp up the nutrient value of your foods.

2. Add lean protein: Consider leaner proteins like chicken, turkey, fish, shellfish, game meats, and eggs. Don't forget tofu and legumes. When choosing beef or pork, opt for grass-fed, organic, or lean cuts to avoid unwanted hormones and excessive animal fat, which may lead to insulin resistance. In this case, it's better to pay more.

3. Avoid dairy: Dairy is often a pro-inflammatory agent, and frequently, non-organic milk has added hormones due to the type of feed given to the cows.

4. Avoid soy: Soy by itself is a good protein source. However, I would be remiss if I did not mention that non-fermented soy can potentially suppress your thyroid function. This is not to say never eat it. Just be mindful of your hormonal balance, and don't eat soy every day. Fermented soy products, like natto and fermented tofu, can be healthy. Also, if you're vegan and only rely on soy as a protein source, take a break and nibble on other plant sources of protein during that time.

5. Sip on nutrients: Spend time in nature and soak in natural light. Research shows that sunlight boosts your vitamin D intake, which can balance your hormone levels.

6. Munch on healthy fats: Omega-3 fatty acids and omega-6 fatty acids are essential in maintaining a healthy body. However, do not make the mistake of counting all fat as "bad" fat to be avoided. Types of healthy fats are omega-3 fatty acids from fish, oils from grass-fed animals and nuts, avocado, coconut, and organic (extra virgin) olive oil.

7. Consume water, tea, and bone broth: Drink plenty of water

throughout the day, make some bone broth, and sip on healing pure celery.

8. Be mindful of glycemic index: High insulin levels can increase your risk of heart disease, diabetes, hypertension, and depression. Reducing sugar and processed carbs in your diet is not enough. Let's say you're munching on pizza every day. As shown in this study, you can improve your lipid profile by replacing refined grains (the basis of your pizza, most likely) with whole grains and other components of the Mediterranean diet!

9. Count your carb consumption: Consider the amount and type of carbs you are consuming. Low-glycemic-index carbohydrate sources (listed below) have the added benefit of being nutrient-dense, which can help reduce inflammation associated with PCOS. The goal is to fill your plate with non-starchy vegetables according to their low or medium GI score.

10. Aim for smaller portions more often: The goal is not to undereat calories but to moderate the spikes in your insulin levels. Eat something small every three to four hours to maintain balanced sugars and prevent unhealthy food overconsumption.

11. Avoid feasting on sugar: There are many natural options for individuals with PCOS regarding sweeteners. These can easily replace granular sugar and are packed with nutrients and beneficial compounds that lower blood sugar levels, improve insulin sensitivity, are anti-inflammatory, and are advantageous to the gut flora. You can always use inulin (like SweetLeaf organic stevia) instead of sugar to counterbalance the sweetness and create a balanced flavour profile for a healthier alternative to sugar.

2.2. Foods to Include and Avoid

Eating healthy foods can help you manage your PCOS and reduce symptoms. This means avoiding foods high in refined sugars, saturated fats, and carbohydrates and choosing nutrient-rich, high-fiber foods. Avoid processed or preserved foods and choose whole foods instead. To improve your overall health when you have PCOS, consider these tips below, which focus on whole, unprocessed foods and lean protein sources.

Foods to include: healthy fats, including avocados, almonds, and olive oil. High-fibre vegetables and fruits, such as calciferous vegetables (broccoli and cauliflower), leafy greens (lettuce and spinach), and berries. Lean protein: focusing on healthy plant-based protein options. Functional foods, such as turmeric and ginger, can help lower inflammatory actions in the body. Probiotics: Provide up to a cup or more each of dark, leafy greens every day, as well as a few servings of live, cultured, and active yogurt each week. Cinnamon and chromium: for their insulin-sensitizing effects, aim for a 1/2 to 1 teaspoon of cinnamon per day, as well as a few servings each day of whole grains, leafy green vegetables, and eggs. Omega-3 fatty acids, including fish oil or flax seeds. Remember that your doctor or nutritionist may adjust the recommended portion sizes if you have calorie restrictions.

2.3. Meal Planning and Portion Control

What's essential in any dietary plan is to eat set portions of foods at the appropriate times to prevent triggering your body to store fat and to help keep blood sugar levels steady. The biggest secret to weight control is to eat small portions of protein, low-GI carbohydrates, and healthy fats combined in every meal and every snack. Despite this knowledge, portion distortion can cause women with PCOS to consume as many calories as their slimmer peers, who are unfortunately not in a "weight-raising" dynamic thinning environment. Even women with PCOS who shed weight often fall prey to the weight-raising siren's call by becoming ravenous. To maintain their weight loss motivation and their new "lifestyle" rather than "dieting" slimmer friends, women with PCOS have to eat throughout the day in a portion-controlled manner. Coach your mind and willpower to put less and more often in your dish.

Meal planning for women with PCOS is most straightforward when they know that eating a small portion of protein combined with slow-burning carbohydrates will keep them feeling full. Skipping carbohydrates will help with weight loss goals but can dramatically increase hunger and possibly vitamin C deficiencies. So eat small protein portions. Small means the same size as a deck of cards for every meal. This portion will minimize cholesterol and the animal-based saturated fat in your diet. Of course, if you are a vegetarian or waving a red flag at red meat, you should choose the exact volume measurement of a non-fat or soy-based higher protein item. Your question might be, "But what is my carbohydrate portion size?" Small! It is not portion-ridden generous servings that exceed small lunch plates as they display in restaurants or on your twelve-inch dinner plates. For women with PCOS, it is two tiny teaspoons, three times daily, within a lifestyle your body will love—the assumption that vegetables should be eaten in more significant portions than fruit needs to be qualified. Fruits contain various vitamins, and we all know that girls want to have fun, but only if they can prevent insulin spikes. Try eating two small teaspoons of fruit two times daily. For your evening snack, eat grapes instead of a cookie because both produce the same blood glucose level.

3

3. Physical Activity and Exercise

Incorporating regular physical activity is crucial to the long-term management of PCOS. Exercise can profoundly improve insulin sensitivity, help maintain a healthy weight, decrease inflammation, manage stress, and reduce androgen levels. Exercise contains the same benefits as healthy dietary changes, producing significantly more favourable results in combination. However, excessive physical activity may have the opposite effect and lead to further reproductive and metabolic disturbances.

Exercise can also have a positive impact on reproductive hormones and weight. Since PCOS is often associated with insulin resistance, which can then lead to unintended weight gain, exercise should be an essential part of PCOS management. Because leptin levels often reflect body fat levels, losing weight may reduce leptin levels, which may help regulate the hypothalamic-pituitary-ovarian axis. Lowering leptin levels may also result in improving menstrual cyclicity. It does not have to be hours spent at the gym to shed excess pounds; 150 minutes per week of moderate weight-bearing activity can make all the difference. The amount of activity required for weight loss varies and is believed to occur with moderate and high activity levels. Keep exercising if you lose weight after exercising regularly for several weeks. Reducing elevated insulin levels may improve serum androgens, cholesterol profiles, and insulin resistance. The three best ways to speed up your metabolism are eating a small, healthy breakfast, eating small meals every three to four hours, and exercising regularly. The goal of participating in a regular exercise program should be to improve insulin sensitivity.

3.1. Benefits of Exercise for PCOS

Do you want to find a natural way to increase feel-good hormones, reduce insulin resistance, and improve fertility? Forget the chocolate cake. Start exercising! The best exercise of all for ovarian and adrenal health is high-intensity interval training. If you're new to exercise, welcome to the beginning of the rest of your life. Change for the better. Starting with a walk is a great way to begin. Increase the pace when you're comfortable. Strength training twice a week combined with 3-5 sessions of 20 minutes of aerobic cardio should make your body happy. Keep in mind that more is not always better. A workout that lasts longer than 40 minutes can increase your cortisol levels, contributing to insulin resistance and weight gain. Remember to enjoy the exercise, too; make time for fun and games.

Exercise in Women with PCOS. The benefits of exercise are awe-inspiring for women with PCOS. The improvement of insulin sensitivity, the long-term increase in insulin receptors, and the lowering of the body's glucose requirements are enough reasons to go on the following day's workout. But if that isn't enough, how about a quicker reduction of stress hormones? Exercise stimulates neurochemical pathways that antagonize the neurohormones released under stress. Whether fighting or flying, you are in better shape when you exercise following an acute stressor. These stress hormones won't increase circulating glucose levels when walking briskly in the park. Improved fertilization rates and embryo quality all add to the importance of exercise. A better night's sleep, improved libido reliability, lower hyperandrogenism, and regulation of the menstrual cycle all benefit women with PCOS. Not only will you look better, feel better, and improve the number on the scale, but you will also feel the goodness from within.

3.2. Creating a Sustainable Exercise Routine

The ecosocial perspective promotes factors consistent with the living being, considering individual differences and group behaviour. The development process takes place through interaction with the social and natural environment.

In PCOS, physical activity has been proven to improve insulin sensitivity cholesterol levels, and alleviate symptoms. Also, according to research, physical activity not only helps manage signs and symptoms but also improves your chances of a healthier future, so it is crucial to aim to exercise regularly to be able to create a sustainable and achievable fitness routine.

If you are new to exercise, starting slowly with easier-level workouts can give you an idea of what your body is capable of. Trying to do a strenuous workout right away can overwhelm you and cause you to slip into a repetitive habit cycle. You are more likely to sustain your fitness routine by feeling comfortable and not highly pushed. Start with a workout routine that is easy to start and maintain. With almost endless exercise opportunities, you are more likely to find a couple of them added to your week. At least three to five days a week are marked off for physical exercise. When choosing activities, also be sure to wear the proper athletic outfit so you can avoid the typical physical obstacles of exercise.

4

4. Stress Management Techniques

Stress management should be an essential part of coping with one's PCOS, especially when stress is seen to trigger increased hormone levels that exacerbate symptoms of polycystic ovarian syndrome. Managing stress is also about taking the time to relax, rest, and take a breather from a demanding lifestyle. Are you nurturing a hobby? Do you make time for yourself? Do you have a mental health day' off from work regularly? These are the questions that you can ask yourself to see if you're doing what is best to manage stress.

- Take time out for fun and relaxation.
- Schedule quiet time alone.
- Listen to your body's and your heart's desires.
- Express yourself.
- Make a list of affirmations and keep them visible.
- Exercise regularly.
- Use relaxation exercises to reduce physical tension.
- Don't do everything; prioritize, and be bold and delegate.
- Use your support network of friends and family.
- Make time for yourself.

- Set some realistic goals, and don't try to be all things to all people

4.1. Understanding the Link Between Stress and PCOS

One piece of the PCOS puzzle that a lot of people glaze over is the role that high levels of stress play in this syndrome. When we are under high-stress levels, our cortisol levels are high. After all, cortisol is the hormone our body produces that helps us effectively deal with seemingly unending stressful situations. However, when these high cortisol levels are sustained for long periods, it causes our body to suppress other essential hormones. According to Dr. Lara Briden, high levels of cortisol release cause a luteinizing hormone (LH) surge. High levels of luteinizing hormone stimulate androgen production, which can lead to signs and symptoms of PCOS.

Fight or flight mode causes our body to suppress other essential hormones, like estrogen and progesterone. Stress was always intended to take over and consume our brains to help us get out of troubled situations, not to be sustained 24/7. That is exhausting for the brain to handle. Essentially, because we are under high levels of stress, other vital hormones our bodies need to function every day are being held hostage. It is easy to understand the link between this and a hormone-imbalanced condition like PCOS. Women with PCOS tend to have higher levels of both chronic and acute stress than women who do not have PCOS. It is also worth noting that a poor response to stress also worsens the symptoms of PCOS. To put it as bluntly as Dr. Lara Briden, the root of the problem in PCOS is the response that our body has to stress. 7

4.2. Mindfulness and Meditation Practices

We live in a hasty, noisy, and highly transacted world. This often leads to chronic stress, especially for women with PCOS who are already stressed out due to hormonal imbalances. When stress becomes chronic, it can lower immunity, worsen PCOS symptoms, and negatively affect our mental well-being. Stress is a part of our lives, and escaping from it is impossible, so to ensure we keep our overall health in check, practicing mindfulness and meditation can significantly reduce our body's stress signals, increase the relaxation response, reduce insulin resistance, reduce androgen support, and help reduce anxiety and elevate mood. Taking time each day to meditate, even for 15 minutes, can be beneficial and bring a sense of calmness and mindfulness. Incorporating mindfulness activities into our daily routine allows us to stay mindful and commence a usable meditation at any time, anywhere, and in any situation.

Be present when meeting, eating, exercising, walking, and talking to others. Most importantly, take the time to savour your food when you eat. Try having regular weekly "power" breaks—taking 5 to 10 minutes to focus on your breath with your eyes closed and attending to your breathing or meditating. Practice gratitude. Keeping a gratitude journal where you write down at least five things you are grateful for each day or setting intentions for the day and reflecting on them through guided meditation can significantly increase positive emotions and life satisfaction. Attend mindfulness or meditation workshops. Use mindfulness or meditation apps. Try it and see how it benefits you and your mental well-being.

4.3. Breathing Exercises and Relaxation Techniques

Are you waking up in the morning feeling exhausted, drained, and overwhelmed, as if you haven't slept all night? Do you find it hard to fall asleep at night? Is your jaw clenched while sleeping? Do you sleepwalk? Or do you suddenly get into emotional rages? Finals are coming up; lots of assignments? And backache problems from long hours of sitting, seriously studying, and typing away?

Just as exercise helps to manage blood sugar levels, relaxation helps to support improved control over your health and well-being. Deep breathing and muscle relaxation can help ease your way to a stress-free mind and life with little effort. Both of these techniques can serve as a reminder of the importance of deep relaxation for overall good sleep at night. As a result, they are effective.

Incorporate these exercises to enjoy the lifetime benefits in many different areas, such as exercising to experience the benefits of being fully relaxed. It is impossible: jumping, hiking, and mountain climbing. Similar to a deep break point, every muscle begins to break point and remains unused. Just as nature has equipped our bodies to erupt from dangers, the chemicals produced within us also have mechanisms to promote this balance. We become more stress-prone to our minds and health.

4.4. Sexual Health, Pleasure, and Wellness Exploration

PCOS can have a significant impact on sexual health and pleasure, affecting libido, vaginal lubrication, and sexual satisfaction. In this chapter, we explore the complexities of PCOS-related sexual dysfunction and provide tips for improving sexual health and pleasure. From open communication with your partner, which plays a crucial role in promoting a satisfying and fulfilling sexual relationship, to exploring different types of sexual activity that can bring pleasure and intimacy, there are various ways to navigate the challenges posed by PCOS. Additionally, incorporating sex toys and other innovative forms of sexual expression can open up new avenues of pleasure and enhance sexual experiences. By embracing your sexuality and acknowledging its importance to your overall well-being, you can reclaim pleasure as an integral part of your journey toward optimal health and self-fulfillment.

5

5. Sleep Hygiene and PCOS

In a constantly awake world due to our highly digitized environment, getting a good night's sleep can be rare. We should have about 6 to 8 hours of sleep every night to maintain general wellness and health. These hours allow the body to regain its ability to function correctly. This is also when we detoxify our bodies and organs through a good night's sleep.

For women with PCOS, lack of sleep increases insulin resistance. This can be bad news. If you're already insulin resistant and have type 2 diabetes, this can make your blood sugar rise quickly. Additionally, growth hormones don't surge in the morning. This hormone is essential for muscle development and repair and the overall management of fat metabolism. Because of this, you tend to accumulate more body fat. On a daily basis, excess fat can add up to 1-2 pounds of weight gain each week.

Exercising at least 2 hours a day decreases these effects, but is just not possible in the hustle and bustle environment. So, monitor your hours of sleep. Practice sleep hygiene by avoiding coffee or any caffeinated products, avoiding foods that have high sugar content during dinnertime, and avoiding overeating food incredibly very close to bedtime. Usually, after 8 p.m., it is considered an excellent time to avoid food. Try to sleep better at night so that you feel great in the morning, too. Engage in activities that can help you relax, such as reading or engaging in meditation exercises. Also, aromatherapy oils, such as lavender and chamomile-based oils, are available to help you relax and fall asleep.

5.1. Importance of Quality Sleep for Hormonal Balance

Sleep is an essential element to health and well-being for both men and women living with PCOS and, in fact, for everyone. Without sound, restful, restorative-quality sleep, you cannot cope with all the demands of the day. Unfortunately, most women living with PCOS do not get enough sleep, as the effects of sleep apnea, OSA (obstructive sleep apnea), or CSA (central sleep apnea) are common health problems that occur in a variety of medical conditions, some of which are more prevalent in women than men. Between pregnancy and menopause, however, many of these conditions are unique to women. Whether these disorders reflect sex-specific influences on respiratory control or occur in the setting of other hormonal and morphologic changes unique to women is unknown.

Indeed, hormonal influences on sleep and breathing may underlie the sex differences in sleep-disordered breathing during different physiologic states of a woman's life. These physiologic states of sleep (both the reproductive and postmenopausal periods) are accompanied by marked changes in the serotonin pathway, the norepinephrine pathway, and other neurotransmitter systems. Sleep disturbance is common in these states and is often related to vasomotor symptoms, nocturnal hot flashes, and sleep-disordered breathing. Because serotonin plays a role in regulating ventilation, sleep, and behavioural state, there are also essential implications of hormonal changes on the ability of these pathways to modulate serotonin drive, especially during reproduction. Hormonal treatment, potential interactions between hormones and arousal states, and potential interactions between menopause and the aging/spontaneous resolution of hormone-related breathing problems are areas where future research is needed.

5.2. Tips for Improving Sleep Hygiene

Avoid bright lights like smartphones, laptops, iPads, etc., within 2 hours of bedtime. If this is not possible, you can use blue light-blocking sponsors to prevent your exposure to the lights and melatonin suppression. Blue light is much more potent than any other light.

Block noise and light using blackout curtains, earplugs, or white noise machines. Follow a regular sleeping routine by sleeping and waking up simultaneously every day, including weekends. This will train your body to wake up and sleep at the right time.

Remove large meals, caffeine, or alcohol at least 3 to 4 hours before bed. These may delay your body's natural release of melatonin, make it hard for your body to relax, and possibly make you wake up several times.

Wind down. Try to stick to activities that make you relax and reduce stress. You can read a book, take a warm bath, or meditate.

Keep your bedroom cool. The room temperature ideal for sleeping is 60°F to 69°F. Technology devices, mattresses, pillows, and your body heat can elevate your room temperature. This may also cause you to have a restless night.

Be aware of hidden sleep thieves in your room. Ensure that no electric appliances are producing noise, light, or heat, interrupting your sleep. You can also cover up the lights on your electronic devices and shut them down or put them on silence. Shut off the clocks that can leave you anxious about how little longer you can sleep before your alarm goes off.

Ideally, wake up in the morning with the sound of the sun and use natural light to help wake up the right way and at the right time. Also, create an ideal bedtime routine by shutting down your bedroom lights and switching to a different schedule for exercise, caffeine, and other stimulating activities earlier in the day. This will give your adrenaline time to drop before you go to bed.

Focus on these helpful and practical suggestions before resorting to sleep aids, as they can potentially become highly addictive and have a detrimental impact on your overall well-being and health. Taking a proactive approach to improving your sleep hygiene and adopting healthy sleep habits will help you address any underlying sleep issues and promote long-term, restful sleep without relying on potentially harmful medications. By implementing these suggestions, you pave the way toward achieving a more fulfilling and rejuvenating sleep experience that positively influences your daily life.

5.3. Establishing a Bedtime Routine

According to a study at Tufts University School of Medicine, having a regular bedtime can be crucial for your health. Irregular sleep patterns can disrupt the body's internal systems and put you at a higher risk of developing chronic disorders. Research is also showing that a lack of sleep and a disruption of the circadian system can increase your chances of developing breast cancer or make you more susceptible to other, more malignant cancers.

The typical guideline for a good night's sleep is 7 to 8 hours of sleep each night. The best way to set a routine is to set a regular bedtime. This gets the body into a routine and helps you mentally prepare your body and mind so that it's time to go to sleep. You must establish that the bed is only for sleep, with a calming nighttime routine to relax you. Relaxing when you get to bed can help you fall asleep faster and stay asleep. Even if you have PCOS or other health issues, a good night's sleep routine can help defend you against breast cancer and other diseases. Although it may take some time, following a regular schedule can help regulate your body's internal balance.

6

6. Supplements and Herbal Remedies

Chromium, zinc, magnesium, essential fatty acids, and numerous other vitamins and minerals are all required by the body in addition to a healthy diet. These are either not fully delivered to the female body when sick with PCOS, or the total absorption of these nutrients from the ingested food is not possible. As a result, many women with PCOS are exposed to a greater risk of mineral deficiencies and, consequently, a greater risk of developing various symptoms of metabolic disorders. Research has shown that the condition is somewhat improved somatically in women with PCOS who opt for supplementation with numerous different nutritional supplements. It may also be possible to reduce individual symptoms by selectively supplementing some minerals and vitamins (for instance, iodine or magnesium).

If you still come across controversial scientific debates on the topic of PCOS, the consensus is clear about decreasing PCOS symptoms through regular physical activity. Regular, daily physical activity is the first 'therapy' for minor menstrual cycle disorders in the majority of healthy women. Overall lifestyle changes, including balanced meals, less calorie-dense food, and regular physical activity, are ultimately part of primary therapy for women with PCOS. Physical activity will contribute to a better outlook on life, among many other health and social benefits. Other benefits of regular physical activity include minimizing the duration of an existing pregnancy, participating in group activities, taking or losing weight, and generally being free of pain, water, dress size, weight loss, and gaining physical strength.

6.1. Key Supplements for PCOS Management

Critical supplements for PCOS management, as already highlighted, and lifestyle modification teamed with superior nutrition support are seen as the first and foremost recommendable treatment approaches for women with PCOS. This section briefly discusses the best-researched dietary supplements clinically proven to ameliorate the underlying physiological issues identified with PCOS and metabolic syndrome. If you found using or eating whole foods beneficial to your overall health, remember to stay with this health regimen. Tea and a small amount of dark chocolate or beautiful red berries are noble sources of polyphenols. Other top polyphenol sources are whole grains, apples, oranges, and darker grapes. For a PCOS condition, you may also use a green tea supplement for its polyphenol capacity and quench your cravings with a small daily serving of dark chocolate or the occasional small serving of 100% chocolate. Uncategorized chronic inflammation is a considerable concern in women with PCOS, where foods with moderate polyphenol content, including turmeric, cherries, green tea, etc., are linked to reduced inflammation. Polyphenol supplements are not expected. Let us remember that food is still the best way to consume polyphenols.

At this stage, Omega 3, the fatty acid of fish oil, is the MVP boyfriend of PCOS. It not only effectively improves insulin resistance, PCOS-relevant inflammation, triglycerides, and LDL cholesterol but also improves depression, which is frequently related to PCOS. In conclusion, Omega 3 is beneficial for many PCOS symptoms. High-quality fish oil is necessary and valuable for PCOS. Omega 3 from fish-in supplements seems more useful than EPA or DHA supplements. High and safe doses of up to 3000 mg EPA+DHA daily, in consultation with your healthcare provider when mindful, might be necessary. Safe daily multivitamins or prenatal vitamins include the whole spectrum of essential B vitamins, including B12, B6, and Bc/Folate, which are significant for PCOS management. Researchers have found that multi-species solid human probiotics reduce insulin resistance and decrease difficult and damaging stomach bacteria. We do not have clear guidance on PCOS-featured probiotic bacterial hours.

However, we realize that the study supports a probiotic, a combination of at least two strains of Rhamnosus, Lactobacillus acidophilus, and Bifidobacterium presented in 200 billion CFUs daily. In addition, other anti-inflammatory, stomach-part-associated strains, such as L. reuteri and, to some extent, lactobacilli and Bifidobacteria, are introduced for many PCOS patients. 100% r-lipoic acid, existing in common, offers dominant stabilization, anti-inflammatory, and weight loss benefits to your PCOS management strategy. (Equal proportions of the r- and S-forms of lipoic are undecided and not recommended because the r- and S-form antagonists hate each other.) More than a healthy, high-fat, fish-centred Mediterranean diet has been reviewed and tested in relation to general diets related to feces and gut flora and positively associated with markers of a healthy gut. High potassium consumption reduces chronic heart disease and some cancers. Adding high body potassium can lower blood pressure, improve bone density, and diminish the loss of muscle and kidney stones. PCOS women can be considered to be high-potassium foods.

6.2. Natural Remedies to Support Hormonal Health

1. Water-dispersible vitamin E. The use of oral estrogen increases the need for vitamin E. Use it in water-dispersible form; start with 50% of its RDA (15 mg) and gradually increase up to 100%. A woman taking plenty of whole grains and plant foods likely gets enough vitamin E from her diet.

2. Freshground flax seed: Flax seeds are a rich source of lignin, which is vital in ablating excess estrogen. Research evidence suggests a 25-gram portion per day.

3. Licorice (Glycyrrhiza glabra). This plant is known to have hormonal activity and has been traditionally used to support women through menopause, the menstrual cycle, and depression. Since it increases cortisol production and is generally not safe to take for long,

4. Dong Quai (Angelica sinensis). Dong Quai is an anti-spasmodic that has a balancing effect on the female hormonal system. Due to its blood-thinning properties, it increases the effects of anticoagulants. It is avoided for heavy period bleeders and during pregnancy.

5. Fenugreek (Trigonella foenum graecum). Fenugreek has a warming effect and is used to relieve the physical and emotional symptoms of the menstrual cycle. It has a blood sugar-lowering effect and is used to stimulate milk production.

6. Pearl powder. It is considered a precious herb in traditional Chinese medicine. It is considered safe to take during pregnancy but in moderation. It is used as a kidney tonic and is supposed to be good for female hormones and emotional well-being.

7. Healthy Habits for Skin and Hair Care

Women want to be confident. Despite the PCOS, they opt to look good. Young and pretty skin, a glowing face, and strong, shiny hair are attributes of good appearance that every woman wishes for. Healthy skin needs to be adequately cleaned; diet and hydration are essential. Proper and regular hygiene is a sign that we care for ourselves and have good hygiene. Do not overuse soaps and detergents on your face. Clean it gently and softly, and pat it dry. Using traditional herbal beauty products can be a good option. Shea butter provides calcium, a rich source of vitamin E, which improves the skin. The right fats are good because they enable the body to absorb fat-soluble vitamins A, D, E, and K. Good fats are also good for your hair. Correct fats in your diet, possibly in dried fruit, eggs, olives or olive oil, and spinach, will give your hair a good look. Carefully rinse off the shampoo from your hair. An excess amount of shampoo can make your hair dry and add washing-wearing tears to the hair as well. Avoid vigorous brushing, as it can cause hair loss. Anxiety also causes hair loss. Keeping your hair clean and stress-free with gentle hands can do a lot to make it luxurious. Regular exercise, yoga, and meditation can all give you the spirit of body wellness and remove your mind from concerns about skin and hair problems. Drink enough water. It is important to keep your body hydrated. Eat more fruits and vegetables. Nourishing food leads to nourishing skin. You are starting today!

7.1. Skincare Tips for Acne and Hirsutism

PCOS is always associated with skin manifestations like acne, hirsutism, and alopecia. It is a severe blow to the self-esteem of women who have been plagued by weight woes. Here are a few skincare tips for acne and hirsutism:

Tip #1: Consult a dermatologist for proper diagnosis and treatment. The dermatologist should prescribe the right products for your skin. Then, one can see improvement after continuous use. Be sure to follow the prescribed medications the dermatologist gave and discuss adding a multivitamin supplement for additional support if needed. Choose beauty products that do not have oily or too-milky formulations as much as possible.

Tip #2: Clean your face regularly. Always cleanse the skin in the morning and night to support overall pH balance. Use a gentle and foaming wash.

Tip #3: After washing, put on a toner immediately. Use a toner to cleanse, just like the Clean & Refreshing Toner, which is ideal for acne-prone skin. Tone or apply acne moisturizing lotion to affected parts of the face or all over your face. It promotes hydration while reducing excess oil and redness on your skin. During the day, wear at least SPF 30 sunscreen to protect the skin from further damage.

Tip #4: Do not pick at your skin. This promotes unwanted scars and potentially acne pitting, which are difficult to change later.

7.2. Hair Care Strategies for Thinning Hair

Hair loss is one of the most common and distressing symptoms of patients with PCOS. It occurs when hair is lost from areas where head hair used to grow. Women with PCOS may notice that their hair loss is unique. Both ends of the affected hairs are often sawn off and thinner than the hair that remains. It can be frustrating because nothing can be done to alleviate the situation due to the state of the body's health. However, it is not necessary to worry, as you can find valuable details in our sample women's healthy hair care guide. Hair restorations, medications, and helpful solutions can also fast-track your beauty. The following are some hair treatment options that may prove beneficial to women with PCOS: low-dose birth control packages, which could help avoid birth control; anti-androgen pills; and hair waves, based on a study published by the American Hair Loss Administration, which belongs to women with PCOS. Patients with PCOS may also practice the volunteer hair care guide below to facilitate further hair loss.

Several topical oils found in clinical trials can promote propagation between terminal hair follicles (when hair loss occurs for a long time), so they are encouraged for patients with hair loss. A blend of 3% rosemary oil plus dilution in a 1% solution after seven months of application was only approved by minoxidil in an experimental sample of 100 people. 87% had increased the follicular fish for triple concentration. During the continuous period, 23% of men applying minoxidil regularly saw a rise in hair thinning, making liposomal vegetarian helpful oil as well.

7.3. Natural Remedies for Common Skin and Hair Issues

Avoid shampoos that contain a lot of sulphates, silicones, and parabens. Those chemicals are estrogen-disruptive; they affect the structure and function of the brain and other reproductive organs. Try using castor oil to open clogged hair follicles and add some shine and lustre to your hair. Bathe 1 tsp of castor oil with 1 tsp of sweet almond oil and two drops of lavender oil, then rub the oil blend through your hair and wrap your hair with a warm towel for 10–20 minutes before shampooing. To exfoliate your skin, mix salt, sugar, oatmeal, or herbal tea to make a good exfoliant for the skin. Mix with jojoba oil or argan oil for the best exfoliants that will help to enhance the moisture-protective barrier of your skin at the same time. You can also go for home remedies like cucumber, green tea, yogurt, aloe, honey, and sugar.

revive Acne Treatment. This will significantly decrease the appearance of blemishes and acne within just hours of treatment. For sensitive skin, apply a thin layer of overnight treatment as a mask for 10–15 minutes before rinsing off. The treatment will effectively help eliminate the dark spots that usually follow after some active acne or pimples. Acne is formed when the hair follicles are clogged with oil and dead skin cells. Eczema, atopic dermatitis, and psoriasis can make it worse to deal with. Acne in the PCOS would be due to the androgen hormone level increasing and raising the sebaceous gland (an oil gland) which is under the skin to produce more oil, which makes the pore more clogged and prone to acne.

8

8. Maintaining a Healthy Weight

Being overweight increases your body's resistance to insulin's effects, leading to increased blood insulin levels. Having increased blood insulin levels can make PCOS conditions worse. That's why keeping your weight under control is an essential aspect of keeping PCOS symptoms at bay. Losing those extra pounds or kilos will not only keep your symptoms under control but will also help you manage other PCOS health risks and diseases, such as diabetes and high cholesterol.

Here's what you can do. First things first, be committed to changing the life you lead. Remember that big and small things can add up to a lost weight. That's why incorporating small healthy changes, such as reducing salt and sugar intake and making regular exercise a part of your daily routine, will help you achieve your healthy body goals. Get your body moving as often as possible towards a healthier you by incorporating simple, healthy living into your daily life. Choose wisely. You have a choice to be happy and healthy with what you put in your mouth, so next time, make healthier choices. It's time to be committed to a healthier lifestyle. Do it now!

8.1. Weight Management Strategies for PCOS

Managing your weight with PCOS simply means making small lifestyle decisions for healthy living and control of symptoms. As a woman with PCOS, you are more likely to suffer from chronic elevated blood sugar, high blood pressure, high lipid problems, and infertility. This is not a special diet that can cure PCOS, but a balanced approach to helping symptoms and the prevention of other disorders.

This is a well-balanced guide taking the balanced calorie diet root, balanced with meals that stay with you, ensuring an outstanding balance of proteins, good fats, carbohydrates, and iron-rich foods set into guidelines for healthier, stable insulin levels.

To achieve and maintain a healthy weight, healthy eating will modify the food choices you select and the quantity based on that selection. A significant part of weight management, considering diet and exercise, can be maintained by engaging in 30 minutes a day of energetically moderate physical activity. You can find things you can do and enjoy; just take a brisk walk or take the stairs for 15 minutes to start.

An intake of a balanced calorie diet in the amount your body uses and being physically active provides many health benefits, including reduced cardiovascular risks and improved symptoms.

8.2. Setting Realistic Goals and Tracking Progress

Set realistic goals. While it might be tempting to set huge, long-term health goals, it's much better to start with much smaller, more achievable short-term goals. Short-term goals are stepping stones to your long-term goals and can help provide a sense of accomplishment and motivation.

Journal about your progress. One of the most important parts of tracking your goals and progress is to make sure to journal about the process and how you feel. Lack of progress can be disheartening, and documenting setbacks and frustrations might give you a chance to address and resolve them before they develop into significant issues.

Celebrate progress—every bit counts! Every bit of progress is still progress. Even if you didn't make it to the gym for a full cardio workout, doing something every day is helping to build your long-term, healthy routine.

Tracking your progress over time often means looking back at the beginning, but why not also take a "progress shot" photo every few weeks? Seeing a visual comparison side-by-side with your original baseline shows how much progress you've made.

Of course, setting realistic weight and diet goals can be tricky. We often have solid preconceived ideas regarding how much or how fast we should be losing weight and the amount of calories that should constitute a healthy diet, but it is imperative to be patient and listen to your body's actual needs. These are based on hunger cues, not outside suggestions. If you aren't accustomed to paying close attention to these needs, re-training yourself on how to learn them can be a tough challenge and will only happen after a while. Unfortunately, some mainstream diet plans can really alienate these natural feelings and lead to more self-destructive dieting behaviours, which often result in losing weight.

8.3. Healthy Approaches to Weight Loss

Counseling services are provided by registered nutritionists to assess the unique nutritional needs of individuals with PCOS and to give advice on weight loss or weight maintenance. Encourage patients who are overweight/obese to lose weight, but be clear that modest weight losses can still improve metabolic, reproductive, and symptom parameters. Tailor eating plans to accommodate the varying energy requirements of these young women, who range in weight from underweight to morbidly obese. Aim for small changes when discussing change with any client, but be mindful of the fine line between what works as a recommendation and upholding patient autonomy and client-focused empowerment. This notion also applies to polycystic ovarian syndrome and the colourful TM nutrition and activity brochure. Provide a copy of the colourful TM nutrition and activity brochure and review the content with clients.

Urge patients to focus on behavioural modification rather than being overly fixated on the scale because the value of positive behavioural changes is often lost when weight is not lost. Stress the importance of self-monitoring eating and tracking food intake, fluids, and physical activity. Encourage clients to limit sedentary activities, keep intake within budget, and incorporate physical activity into their daily routine. Teach clients about the close relationship between caloric intake and energy output and the need for a minor increase in energy expenditure or decrease in energy intake to lose weight. Discuss a variety of nutrition and activity interventions because no single intervention is effective for all patients with polycystic ovarian syndrome. Promote consumption of predominantly nutrient-rich, low-energy-dense foods. In addition, incorporating the use of artful eating strategies can be beneficial for young adults with polycystic ovarian syndrome who want to manage their caloric intake.

9

9. Fertility and PCOS

I t is pretty difficult to conceive if you have PCOS. When women with PCOS do conceive, one of the most common problems associated with the condition happens during pregnancy. Women with PCOS are known to suffer from infertility. It is not uncommon for women with PCOS trying to get pregnant to go through four or more cycles of fertility treatments to attempt to conceive. Many women with PCOS resort to the use of ovulation-inducing medications (OIMs) to produce mature follicles that are likely to release eggs. Most reports suggest a successful pregnancy rate of up to 60% for clomiphene citrate, which can be as high as 85% combined with metformin (Glucophage).

IVF (in-vitro fertilization) is another option for those wanting to get pregnant. There are clinics all around the country. However, IVF is a costly treatment that can be very taxing on a person's health, and there is no guarantee that conception will take place. The Victorian Assisted Reproductive Treatment Authority states that the success rate of IVF treatments is 30% for fresh transfers and just 21.5% for frozen-thawed transfers in women up to 24 years of age. The success rate diminishes with the increasing age of the woman. Furthermore, there is an opportunity for several babies to be born at the same time, leading to multiple pregnancies. Triplets and other high-order multiples are frequently the result of IVF treatment. However, it is suggested that if a woman gets pregnant using IVF, she should be on a healthy diet to ensure the best chance that both mother and baby are healthy throughout the pregnancy. In addition, it will also ensure that the baby grows the right amount so that it is not "overweight" once born.

9.1. Understanding the Impact of PCOS on Fertility

Some, but not all, women living with PCOS are concerned about their ability to conceive. We constantly hear comments online such as "my infertility" and "having PCOS means you are infertile.". Yes, PCOS can have a severe impact on your ability to conceive, and if you are looking to fall pregnant and are struggling, routines can be a welcome and healing thing. There are heaps of helpful resources that talk about falling pregnant with PCOS that are worth further investigation if this resonates with you, including a hormone tuning guide for fertility. As for us, we would instead take one tiny but all-important step back from saying, "My PCOS caused my infertility.".

This is directly counter to what conventional medical knowledge often suggests. Still, we prefer to look at PCOS not as a condition that causes infertility but instead as a condition that means bodies aren't in a state of health where they can easily fall pregnant if they are looking to do so. Put simply, PCOS doesn't "take babies away." It simply means our body needs a bit more support to help us be healthy or be able to fall pregnant. The strategies recommended will help improve your fertility by supporting your general health.

9.2. Fertility Treatments and Options

If you are trying to conceive, both you and your partner should undergo fertility checks separately. Visiting a fertility specialist can determine whether you have ovulatory dysfunction, and these specialists can assist you through the process of making decisions about fertility treatment options. One consideration is clomiphene citrate (Clomid) therapy and metformin therapy, which will induce ovulation and help eggs start maturing. The patients have about a 20% chance of a live birth rate with twin pregnancies.

Another consideration is gonadotropin injections, in addition to trigger shots, which can help ovulating eggs start maturing. Patients also have about a 22% chance of a live birth rate with twin pregnancies. Controlled ovarian hyperstimulation is an additional fertility treatment that could help ovulatory infertile women or polycystic patients produce multiple mature oocytes. This should be used for patients with tubal damage, diminished ovarian reserve, advanced maternal age, ovarian dysfunction, or endometriosis. The treatment includes ovarian ultrasound and blood work, ovulation monitoring, a hysterosalpingogram as a test for tubal patency, and intrauterine insemination in selected cases. Ovarian hyperstimulation also has a 20–30% live birth rate (with 30–40% for multiple pregnancies and usually less than 5% for higher-order multiples).

9.3. Lifestyle Factors That Support Fertility

One of the most important things women can do to increase their chances of conception is to nourish their systems effectively. At the same time, we need to manage the stress that can be present when we are not in as much control as we would like. The secret to balancing both of these issues is to surround yourself with support. In every area of your life, you need to examine what drains you and what supports you and make the necessary changes. Friends, family, therapists, support groups, and the proper medical treatment can help you through the confusion of infertility treatment.

Consistency is one thing that we need to have in our lives for our biochemistry to work effectively. Consistency in your lifestyle and diet can increase the effectiveness of your fertility treatments, but make sure these changes are ones that you can live with as long-term habits. If you are doing things that are too hard to manage at this time, you will quickly become stressed, and physical stress can be just as detrimental to your condition as a lack of healthy habits.

10

10. Navigating Medical Treatments for PCOS

Navigating medical treatments for PCOS can be difficult, but an open-minded, well-informed approach could bring much-needed benefits in terms of quality of life and control of long-term comorbidities. Opting for lifestyle changes is the first line of treatment recommended by most clinicians. With evidence mounting that supports diet and exercise as effective alternatives or mediators to traditional medications, it's always preferable to lead with the former pair. Nonetheless, symptoms can present as uncomfortable, out-of-the-blue, and very wellness-affecting experiences. Anticipating any trouble from a supportive medical standpoint is always good. Consult with your primary care physician, nutrition specialist, and reproductive endocrinologist about prescription medications in addition to any alternatives you might choose to enlist in your fertility or symptom-elimination cause.

In choosing your care plan, I encourage you to consider the long-term outlook. There is evidence for Type 2 and the increased potential of cardiovascular disease risk with the insulin resistance and hyperinsulinemia of PCOS. Additionally, consider that once full-blown intervention is sought, it is harder to change the metabolic picture and the risks that go with it. The cost and often unnecessary toxicity of additional medication, while often proposable, need to be carefully pondered in the backdrop of a possibly lifelong care plan. And always, always listen to a second opinion! And what a stroke of luck we are living! We have both reproductive endocrinology and functional care. And we don't necessarily need to choose only one!

11

11. Building a Support Network

The importance of a well-balanced support

If you have been newly diagnosed with PCOS, you are going to feel bewildered. If you have been dealing with PCOS for years, you are going to feel frustrated. Both of these are normal feelings associated with PCOS. But it is crucial not to let PCOS isolate you from the rest of the world. PCOS is one of the leading causes of infertility; you are not alone. There are women who share your frustrations and someday will share your victory, women who are going through the same stomach pains after overeating sugar at an office party, and women who mumble to themselves when people ask them, "Have you tried having sex on this day?" PCOS is not a widely recognized syndrome, and because of that, you can feel somewhat distant from everyone else when you barely have time to build a relationship to begin with. This is why creating a supportive and knowledgeable network is vital.

Building a support network

How you structure your network will depend on how you usually socialize. If you are an introvert who is computer illiterate, it will be difficult to go online and build a network. However, if you are really adept at computers, you can find forums in which you can meet and discuss common issues. If you are politically active, look for local organizations that could help you build a network. If you are a closet introvert, a big event with lunches or dinners where they discuss their issues would be helpful for you. If you are in college, you can start a support club on campus. If you are outgoing and want more interesting social support, you can try out for a walk/run marathon sponsored by a PCOS support group. Podcasts and webcasts are also readily available for your comfort. People in a support group have the same feelings as you. This will be a company that you've secretly been looking for but are afraid to ask. Not only will you get information, but you will also get companionship.

11.1. Connecting with Other Women in Similar Situations

Create and thrive with support from family and friends, but also make an effort to connect with other women who are going through similar experiences as you. One way to do that is to join support groups specifically for women living with polycystic ovarian syndrome. With the help of these established groups, you can receive support that only other women in the same situation can understand.

A support group can provide continuous encouragement as you journey along. Setbacks will always be a part of the journey, but a support group can offer continuous encouragement to try one more time or to tackle the next milestone. There are many such groups on Facebook that you can join, with some having members from every part of the world. Others are gender-specific for women only or simply for women who are trying to conceive. Be sure to join a diverse group with members from all walks of life, young and old, and from different backgrounds. Also, consider joining one that has a trained psychologist who can help with the emotional aspects. Some of the support groups will occasionally offer egg-freezing discounts and special forums to share the ovarian tissue-freezing journey

12. Empowering Women to Take Control of Their Health

There is a natural hierarchy in deciding who controls our health. It is the woman whose health depends on it. Sadly, most of them sit like defenceless little girls while their health is handed over to whoever they think can give them the kind of help they need. Most don't realize that the best help in life is free. It is your right to be in charge of your health. This means getting properly informed through personal efforts and having the self-confidence to be actively involved in your health.

I am not a doctor. I do not claim to heal you. All I can do is lay a path for you to follow. An informed path. By taking PCOS under our wing, did you realize that you are now considered a lower insurance risk than women who don't know that they have PCOS? The only condition is to carefully monitor your health by living a healthy lifestyle and correcting imbalances. PCOS connects the pieces of dysfunction in the female body. PCOS is a warning that not everything in the female body is functioning optimally. PCOS is a reminder that you are responsible for your health. It is the female body and the female hormones that ultimately control how healthy you are.

13.3. Encouragement for Continued Self-Care and Wellness

You may have periods when you don't feel well. Don't make things worse by not taking care of yourself because you don't feel well. It is believed that infertility can be stressful. Believe that if you pay attention to caring for yourself, you can decrease the risks of some of the health complications that are associated with PCOS, such as obesity, high blood pressure, heart problems, diabetes, endometrial cancer, and depression. When you pay attention to self-care, you also increase your overall emotional health. Set some positive goals for how you can continue your health care. Doing so has put you on the right path toward good health and wellness. Remember to believe that the health of your body is worth the effort because it is a good investment.

Use these tips to help you take responsibility for your overall self-care and wellness. Remember that you may have to adapt your goals to what is in your best interest and what is realistic for you. Sometimes, setting health and wellness goals harms your emotional health more than good if they are unrealistic. Also, remember that becoming healthier and achieving your wellness goals will not happen overnight. It will take time and patience. But, bit by bit, with hard work, the steps of self-care and wellness will turn into a new lifestyle. Along the way, also remember that patience is one of the many valuable lessons that others can teach you and that can produce great rewards.

12

References

1. Bhalerao A, Aranha I. Polycystic ovarian syndrome (PCOS), distress of female reproductive health. Shanlax International Journal of Arts Science and Humanities. 2021;8(S1-Feb):46-53. researchgate.net

2. Armanini D, Boscaro M, Bordin L, and Sabbadin C. Controversies in the pathogenesis, diagnosis and treatment of PCOS: focus on insulin resistance, inflammation, and hyperandrogenism. International journal of molecular sciences. 2022 Apr 8;23(8):4110. mdpi.com

3. Samish DK, Chapter 6, Role of Diet in Polycystic Ovarian Syndrome (PCOS). Home Science And Extension. 2023. researchgate.net

4. Hmedeh C, Ghazeeri G, and Tewfik I. Nutritional management in polycystic ovary syndrome: challenges and opportunities. International Journal of Food Safety, Nutrition and Public Health. 2021;6(2):120–30. Westminster.ac.uk

5. Dos Santos IK, Ashe MC, Cobucci RN, Soares GM, de Oliveira

Maranhão TM, Dantas PM. The effect of exercise as an intervention for women with polycystic ovary syndrome: A systematic review and meta-analysis. Medicine. 2020 Apr 1;99(16):e19644. lww.com

6. Phimphasone-Brady P, Palmer B, Vela A, Johnson RL, Harnke B, Hoffecker L, Coons HL, Epperson CN. Psychosocial interventions for women with polycystic ovary syndrome: a systematic review of randomized controlled trials. F&S Reviews. 2022 Jan 1;3(1):42–56. researchgate.net

7. Khafagy G, El Sayed I, Abbas S, and Soliman S. Perceived stress scale among adolescents with polycystic ovary syndrome. International journal of women's health, 2020, Dec 29:1253–8. tandfonline.com

8. Daescu AM, Dehelean L, Navolan DB, Gaitoane AI, Daescu A, Stoian D. Effects of Hormonal Profile, Weight, and Body Image on Sexual Function in Women with Polycystic Ovary Syndrome. InHealthcare 2023, May 19 (Vol. 11, No. 10, p. 1488). MDPI. mdpi.com

9. Chantelouve M, Ripoll L. Endocrine disruptors in cosmetics: a review. Molecules, 2022. uqac.ca

10. Chen H, Li J, Cai S, Zeng S, Yin C, Kuang W, Cheng K, Jiang Y, Tao M, Chu C, Hocher JG. Impact of body mass index (BMI) on the success rate of fresh embryo transfer in women undergoing first in vitro fertilization/intracytoplasmic sperm injection (IVF/ICSI) treatment. International Journal of Obesity. 2022 Jan;46(1):202–10. [HTML]

www.ingramcontent.com/pod-product-compliance
Lightning Source LLC
Chambersburg PA
CBHW072341270726
48659CB00023B/2155